The Complete Breastfeeding Book

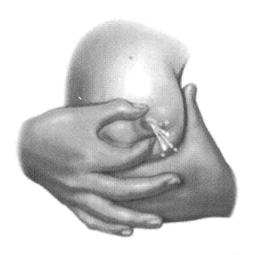

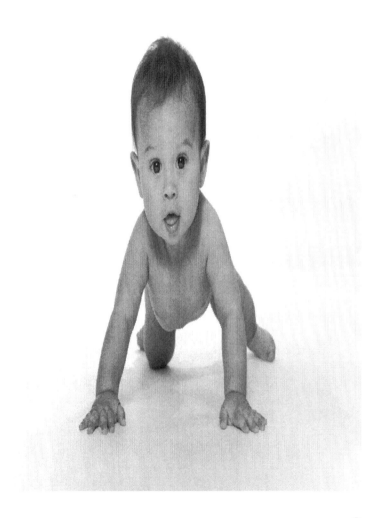

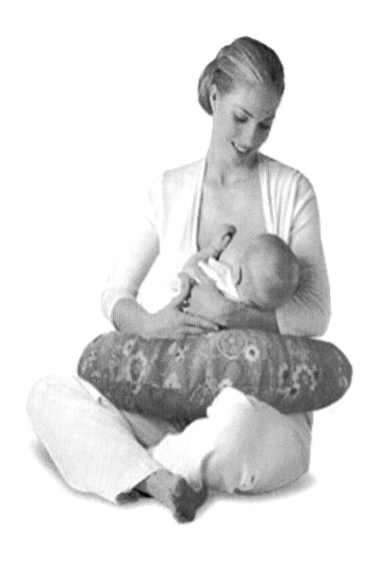

The Complete Breastfeeding Book

*How To Make More Milk
The Ultimate Guide For
Nursing Mothers*

Emma Lockhart

Copyright Notice

Contents

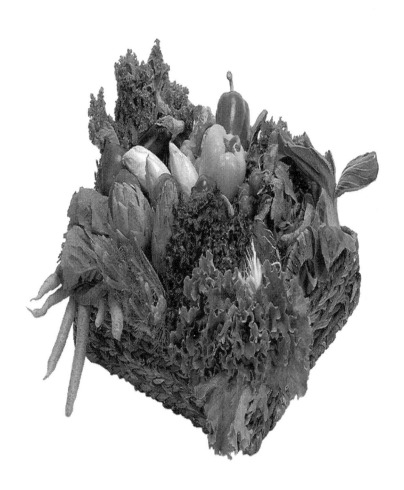

Preface: The Breastfeeding Mindset

B reastfeeding is a great gift for you as well as your infant. Several mothers feel happiness and gratification in the physical and psychological communion they experience with their baby while breastfeeding.

These emotions are augmented by the discharge of the hormones prolactin, which creates a peaceful, nurturing feeling that enables you to relax and concentrate on your baby, and oxytocin, which encourages a sense of love and connection between you and your newborn baby.

These strong feelings may be the explanation why lots of first time mothers who've breastfed their baby choose to breastfeed the children that follow.

Breastfeeding provides health advantages for mothers as well as psychological satisfaction. Generally speaking, women who breastfeed often lose their pregnancy weight faster; about two or three pounds per month. In addition, the hormones oxytocin acts to return the womb to its standard size faster and will reduce postpartum bleeding.

Research demonstrates that women who have breastfed experience lower rates of breast cancer and ovarian cancer later in life.

Some studies imply that breastfeeding your newborn child can result in an increase in bone mineral density after weaning that could protect you against osteoporosis and bone fractures in old age, even though this hasn't been shown conclusively. Breastfeeding delays the return of the mother's menstrual, which can help expand the time between pregnancies.

Breastfeeding can also give an all-natural form of contraceptive if the mother's menses have not returned. Manufacturers of formula continue to refine their goods in effort to spark its attributes as closely as possible, as researchers learn more about the composition of human breast milk.

It's difficult to totally mimic a substance as intricate as human breast milk; however, baby formula does provide an option in instances where it is not possible to breastfeed exclusively or to supply express or donated breast milk in a bottle.

Some new mothers are affected by physical conditions that interfere with breast milk production, like inadequate growth of the glands that produce milk or the impacts of breast reduction surgery.

While few apparent medical problems forbad breastfeeding, you may experience physical or mental resistance to the process.

Nursing your child should not hurt if your infant is latched on to the breast correctly, but incorrect attachment may cause nipple pain as well as bleeding-especially during the very first couple of days of breastfeeding. Some mothers feel deterred by this unfavorable early experience and want to stop breastfeeding.

However, in some cases, a lactation practitioner, nurse or pediatrician is able to help you reposition your infant right at the breast and get breastfeeding off to a much more comfortable start.

New mothers are also often influenced by the advice and experiences of friends and relatives.

In the event your friends or relatives near you did not breastfeed their kids or do not understand its advantages, they may encourage you to stop breastfeeding and feed your child formula as an alternative, I personally do not advise you to choose this option at an early stage of your child's life.

Introduction

They say "breast is best", however, your newborn usually doesn't arrive with a breastfeeding manual. That's where this breastfeeding guide may just come in handy. You want to supply your baby with the best nutrition possible, but might not be aware of things like proper latching techniques or the foods which are best for any breastfeeding mother.

Therefore, here is just about everything you need to know about breastfeeding, from birth to when it's time to wean.

Chapter 1

A Mother's Guide to Breastfeeding

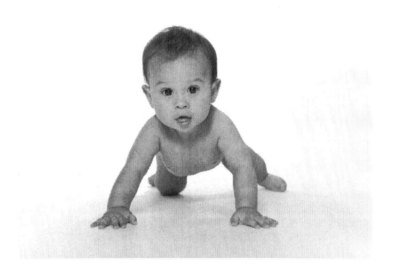

How to produce more nutrition for yourself and your child

To understand the true importance of eating a balanced diet while you are breastfeeding, it's

14

helpful to think of your baby as a sort of symbiotic being. If you take in a sufficient amount of nutrition, then so will they.

However, if your diet is insufficient in nutrients, your baby will fail to receive the vital dietary elements that they desperately need during their first months of life. In addition, poor eating habits can result in a mother's recovery being prolonged and inadequate milk production.

A new mother's dietary requirements are much the same as when she was still pregnant. You are still, essentially eating for two, so you must continue to eat the same amounts and nutritious foods to ensure that you lactate properly and maintain a good supply of milk for your baby.

By not keeping up with this nutrient rich diet, you are jeopardizing not only the quality of your milk, but the amount you have to offer your newborn.

Some important nutritional tips to keep in mind while breastfeeding

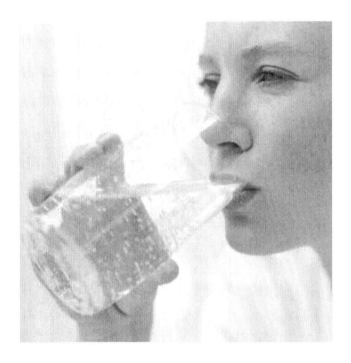

During the time in which you are breastfeeding, you must remember that your diet is your baby's diet. In order for your baby to get the most benefit from your food choices, you have to focus on nutrient rich foods, so that your baby can grow and develop properly. Here are a few things that you should keep in mind while breastfeeding:

- Drink plenty of fluids, but avoid drinking too much water, as it will dilute the breast milk. Instead, consider drinking teas and broths to rehydrate and to keep your breast milk supply adequate for your growing baby.

- Eat smaller meals more often. It's normal for your body to go through a period of adjustment to no longer being pregnant, so you may find that your appetite limps isn't what it used to be. So, ease in your role of new mother and concentrate on eating less more frequently until you become reacquainted with being non-pregnant again.

- If you discover that your baby's bowel movements are slightly different than they should be, then think about what you ate in the last day or so and avoid those foods for a while. Re-introduce them slowly into your diet over time, and pay close attention to how your baby reacts to them again. It could just be that they have to get used to that particular food, or they may even have an allergy to reaction it.

How Proper Nutrition Helps to Build Antibodies

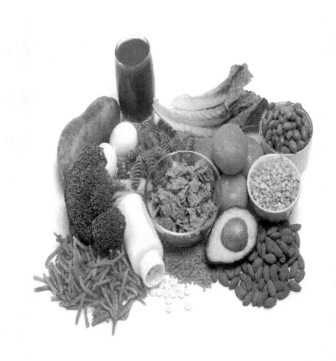

Just as a mother's diet passes from her to her newborn, so do vital antibodies. These antibodies are essential for fending off harmful viruses and other foreign body invaders.

You, having, of course, lived much longer than your child, have had the opportunity to build up antibodies to ward of the common cold or flu, your newborn has not though.

Therefore, they are more prone to becoming sick. However, a mother who has a nutrient rich diet is likely to produce more antibodies, which she can then pass on to her child to prevent them from coming down with any number of ailments during the first months of life.

The best part is that simply maintaining a balanced diet ensures that you will produce enough breast milk and antibodies to help keep your child healthy and happy.

Chapter 2

Healthy Eating Tips for New Mothers

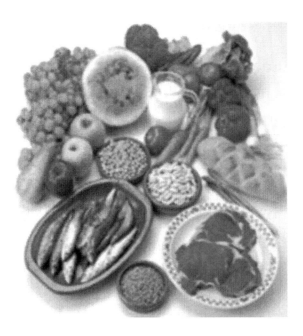

There are a variety of food groups and vitamins that are essential for breastfeeding women. Some women may get all of the important nutrients and vitamins that they need through their diet.

However, if you feel that you don't, you may want to consult with your doctor about the best supplements for you. Here are a few of the important dietary needs that you should consider during your time breastfeeding:

- Get enough vegetables and fruits. Eating plenty of leafy green vegetables, which are high in a number of vitamins and minerals, and fruits, are very important while breastfeeding. Try to buy organic, if possible, but frozen fruits and vegetables will work just fine in fresh options aren't available.

- Don't skimp on the protein. A great source of protein is lean meats and beans, such as lentils or pinto beans, as well as nuts, poultry, cheese, and eggs. It helps us to produce antibodies and hormones, and is necessary for the repair of our cells. However, don't overdo it with the protein, as it is converted to glucose within our systems if consumed in mass quantities.

Carbohydrates

Vitamin A

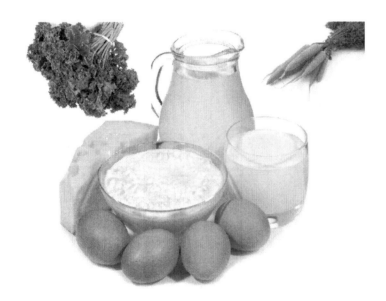

Vitamin A. This vitamin contains retinol and beta-carotene. Both are necessary to maintain healthy respiratory, digestive, and urinary systems. Vitamin A is also vital for good eyesight, and cell division and growth. You can find retinol in liver, dairy products, and eggs. Beta-carotene is found in carrots, mangoes, kale, and spinach.

Vitamin C

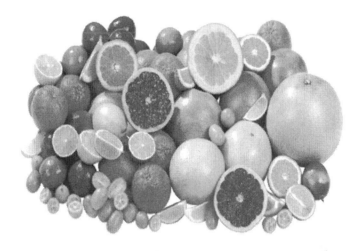

Vitamin C. Assists in absorption of iron, and helps to make certain neurotransmitters, as well as collagen. It is found in citrus fruits, peppers, potatoes, strawberries, and a variety of vegetables.

Vitamin D

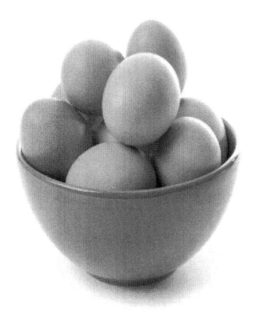

Vitamin D. Aids in healthy teeth and bones, by increasing calcium absorption. It is present in eggs, certain fish (such as tuna and salmon), fish liver oil, and is also produced by exposure to sunlight.

Vitamin E

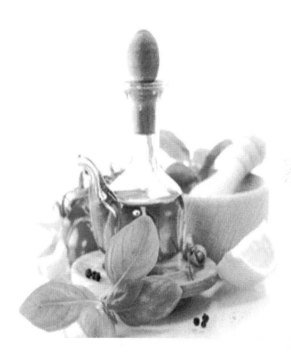

Vitamin E. provides the body with vital antioxidants, and helps the body to fight against certain diseases. It is found in vegetable oils, whit germ, seeds, and margarine.

Vitamin K

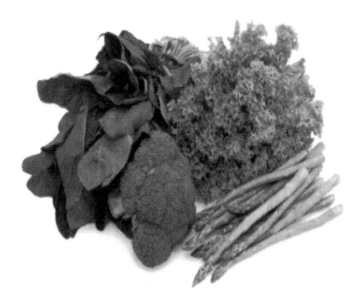

Vitamin K. Assists the body's ability to form proteins and in blood clotting. It is found in green leafy vegetables, such as broccoli and Brussels sprouts.

Thiamin B1

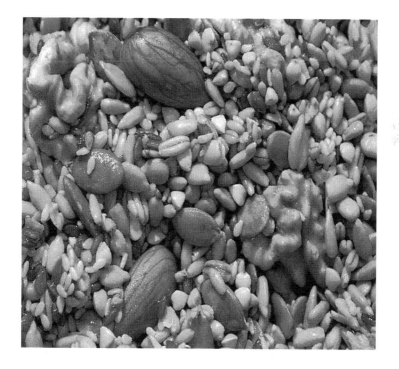

Thiamin (B1). Necessary to obtain energy from carbohydrates, and to prevent the buildup of toxins. It is present in pork, liver, kidneys, and nuts.

Riboflavin B2

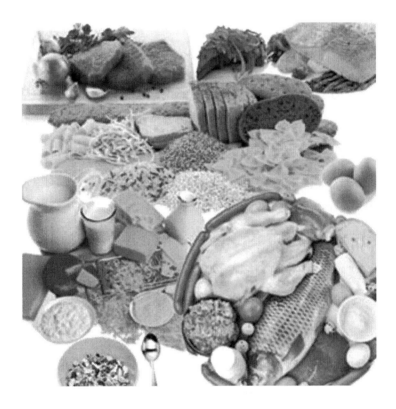

Riboflavin (B2). Is needed to release energy from the food that you eat. It is found in yogurt, meat, poultry, fish, and certain fortified cereals.

Pyridoxine B6

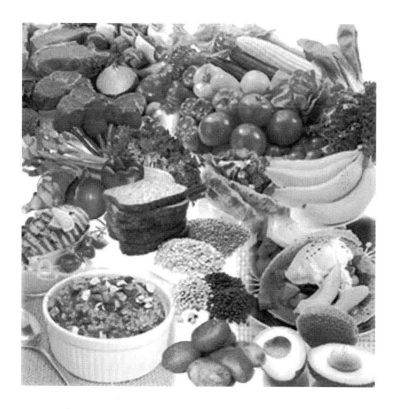

Pyridoxine (B6). Vital to immune function and helps to release energy from the proteins that you eat. It is also important for the formation of red blood cells and for nervous system function. It is found in tofu, whole meal bread, nuts, bananas, lean meats, eggs and poultry.

Niacin

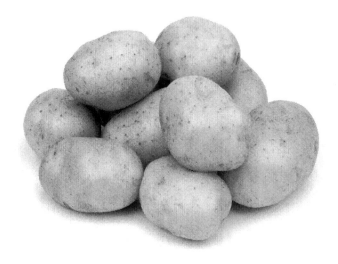

Niacin. Helps you to maintain healthy skin and a digestive system, in addition to producing energy in your cells to form neurotransmitters. It is present in lean meat, poultry, potatoes, nuts, and pulses.

Pantothenic Acid

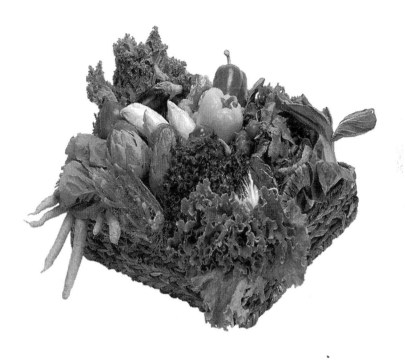

Pantothenic acid. Helps to relieve energy from the food that you eat, and is necessary for synthesis of fat, red blood cells, and cholesterol. It is found in meat, vegetables, liver, dried fruits and nuts.

Biotin

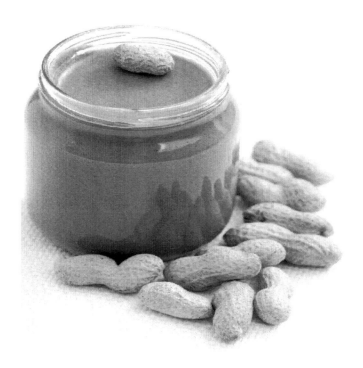

Biotin. Vital in the synthesis of cholesterol and fat. It is present in liver, yeast extract, egg yolk, and peanut butter.

Folic Acid

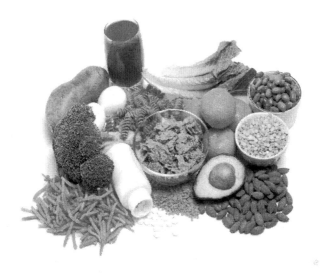

Folic acid. Necessary for cell division and for the formation of proteins, RNA, and DNA. It is present in Brussels sprouts, broccoli, wheat germ, pulses, bread, and fortified breakfast cereals.

Cyanocobalamin B12

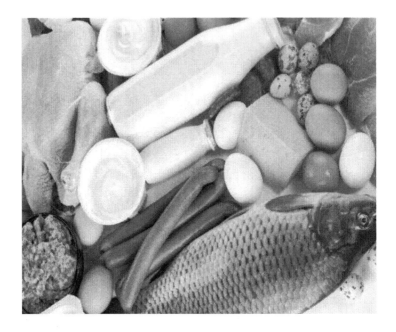

Cyanocobalamin (B12). Necessary for the production of myelin, DNA, and RNA. It is found in meat, poultry, fish, eggs, dairy, and tofu.

Fats

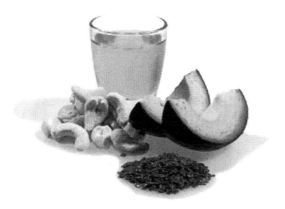

Don't forget the fats. Fats, such as: saturated fats, monounsaturated fats, polyunsaturated fats, and cholesterol, help to maintain healthy skin and body functions.

They are also vital for the production of nerve coatings and cell membranes. They can be found in butter, cheese, fatty meats, and cooking oils.

Macro and Micro Minerals

- **Potassium**. Regulates heart rate and helps to maintain blood pressure. It is found within avocado, fresh or dried fruits, seeds or nuts, bananas, and pulses.

- **Chloride**. Necessary for stomach formation, and to maintain an electrolyte and fluid balance. It is present in foods that contain salt.

- **Calcium**. Helps to build strong bones and healthy teeth, and is important for muscle function and blood clotting. It is found in milk, dairy products, green leafy vegetables, and sesame seeds.

- **Magnesium**. Aids in nerve impulses and muscle contractions, as well as in formation of bones and teeth. It is present in nuts, green vegetables, cereals, and pulses.

- **Sodium**. Regulates your body's fluid balance, and is vital for muscle and nerve function. It is present in processed meats, table salt, yeast extracts, and tinned anchovies.

- **Phosphorous**. Helps to maintain healthy teeth and bones, and is important for the absorption of vital nutrients. It is present in red meat, milk, dairy products, seafood, and whole grains.

- **Zinc**. Helps with growth, immunity and reproduction. It also boosts the power of numerous enzymes. It is found in oysters, nuts, whole grains, beans, and certain seeds.

- **Iron**. Aids in healthy cartilage, gums, and teeth, and is necessary for the production of vital hemoglobin. It is found in kidneys, liver, red meat, egg yolk, sardines, green leafy vegetables, and certain dried fruits.

- **Water**. It is vital for flushing out toxins and re-hydrating the body. It is found in liquids, milk, dairy products, vegetables, and meats, amongst many other things.

Chapter 3

Reasons for Extended Breastfeeding

For many years, researchers have been studying what it is that makes breast milk the perfect food for babies. They found that it contains nearly 200 compounds that help to fight infections, assist in digestion, support brain growth and function, and help to mature the immune system.

These compounds are things that cannot be duplicated by any means other than a mother's milk.

The benefits of long term breastfeeding are numerous for both mother and child. For the baby, the benefits include: decreased risk of asthma, obesity, allergies, as well as some cancers which afflict children. It also has been associated with improving your baby's intelligence, as the nutrients that are found in breast milk aid in brain growth. Breast milk offers your child certain elements which formula does not, and you will probably start to see the benefits of it by the time your baby is around 3 months old.

Breastfeeding for an extended period of time is also good for the mother, as the hormones that breastfeeding produces help to contract your uterus back to its pre-pregnancy size and will prevent increased blood loss directly after giving birth. Also, mothers that practice extended breastfeeding are at a lower risk of being diagnosed with pre-menopausal breast cancer.

By making sure that you breastfeed your baby for as long as possible, you are providing them with the best possible future you can give, and ensuring that their bodies and minds are ready to take on the world.

The Changes Your Body Undergoes Before Breastfeeding

One of the first things a woman notices when they first conceive, aside from a missed period, is tender or swollen breasts. Your bra cup might have suddenly gone up a size or two and your areolas probably darkened. These were the first signs that your body was preparing for breastfeeding while you were pregnant.

The inside of your breasts were undergoing a drastic change, as well. The placenta that was developing triggered the release of progesterone and estrogen, which then stimulated the biological systems that are responsible for lactation.

Supportive tissue and milk glands, as well as fat, has always made up a good portion of your breasts' mass. The truth is that your body, in actuality, had been preparing for lactation even before you were born.

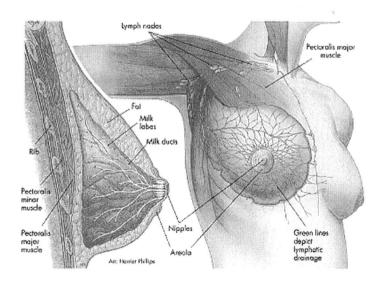

Your milk ducts had already formed while you were in utero, while your mammary glands remained dormant until puberty resulted in hormones which triggered their maturation.

Pregnancy causes those mammary glands to increase their activity. Before your baby is even born, each of your breasts has the potential to be around 1 ½ heavier than they were prior to becoming pregnant, due to glandular tissue taking the place of fat cells.

Within your now swollen breasts is a network of canals which are called milk ducts. Pregnancy hormones caused these ducts to multiply and increase in size, whereby they branched off into smaller channels close to the chest wall, which is the ductless.

At the end of each of these duct channels are small sacs called alveoli. A cluster of alveoli is known as a lobule, and a cluster of lobule is called a lobe. Each of your breasts will contain anywhere between 15 to 20 of these lobes, and there is one milk duct for each lobe.

The alveoli is the milk production site, and it is surrounded by muscles that squeeze the glands in order to force the liquid into the ductless. This ductless leads to an even larger duct that pools milk directly beneath the areola.

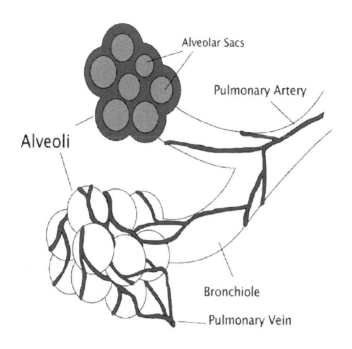

These milk pools are, essentially, reservoirs that store the milk until your baby is ready to feed. Your milk duct system will have probably started to develop around your second trimester, in preparation for your impending arrival, so that you would be able to nourish your child even if they were born prematurely.

Chapter 4

The Benefits of Breastfeeding

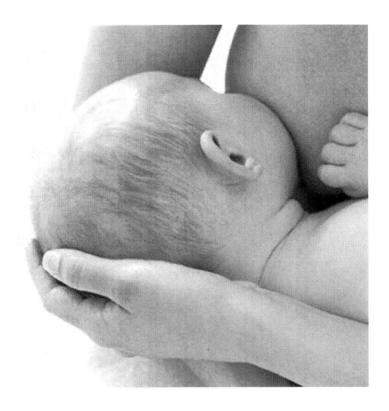

There are a number of benefits to breastfeeding. It is, arguably, the most important thing you can do for your child. It helps to boost their immune system, promotes healthy growth, and, best of all, it's absolutely free. In addition to keeping your grocery bill down, it can also help to lower your medical costs.

Here are a few key reasons why breast is best:

- Breastfed babies get sick less often and their illnesses aren't as severe should they become ill. They are less prone to developing ear and respiratory infections, amongst other things.

Also, the antibodies you transfer to your baby help prevent them from developing allergies. Once your child's immune system develops, they will produce their own antibodies, but for the time being yours will protect them against sensitivities to certain foods.

- Sucking on your breast will help with the alignment of the jaw and help to

45

develop the cheekbones. Therefore, breastfed babies tend to require less orthodontic care when older.

- Breast milk is always available and requires no preparation. It has all of the nutrition your baby needs, so you don't have to worry about spending money on formula to supplement if you produce an adequate amount.

- Breastfeeding will cause the mother to bleed less after birth, as well as return the uterus to its previous shape. In addition, breastfeeding helps you to burn more calories, in order to assist in the shedding of those pregnancy pounds.

- Above all else, breastfeeding provides a bond between mother and child that is truly remarkable. The same cannot be said for formula feeding.

Beginning Breastfeeding

When your baby is first born, it's best to bring them directly to your breast. Though you are not yet producing breast milk, you are producing colostrum that protects your baby against infections. Don't panic if you're baby does not latch on right away, as that is perfectly normal.

Breastfeeding isn't an exact science, as some might think. Practice makes perfect, as well as a whole lot of patience. So, don't hesitate to ask for help from a nurse if you feel you need it. Keep in mind, however, that breastfeeding shooed not be painful. If the latch hurts, then break the latch and try again.

Nursing should be done quite frequently, as more nursing means quicker production of mature milk and larger quantities of it. Aim on breastfeeding for 10 to 15 minutes per breast every couple of hours.

Your baby crying is a sign that they are hungry, so feed them before they even begin to cry. During the first week or two, you might have to wake your baby when it's time to breastfeed.

If he or she has been sleeping for more than four hours, it's a good idea to wake them up and offer the breast. A key thing to remember is that each breastfeeding session can take up to forty minutes, so get comfortable before you begin.

Chapter 4

Positioning During Breastfeeding

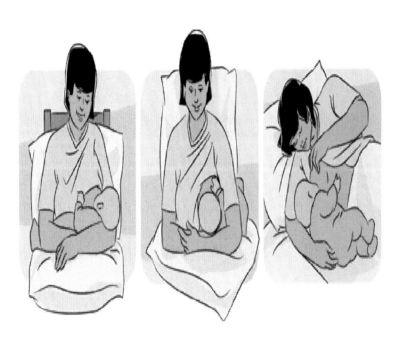

For many women, the act of breastfeeding requires a certain amount of skill, and doesn't come as naturally as it might for others. The trick is in the positioning, as it usually accounts for a good majority of unsuccessful feedings and injured nipples.

You should begin by gently stroking your baby's cheek with your nipple until they latch on. Make certain that the baby gets a mouthful of areola as well as just the nipple. Remember, comfort is key, so make yourself cozy beforehand. Here are the breastfeeding positions that you may find helpful.

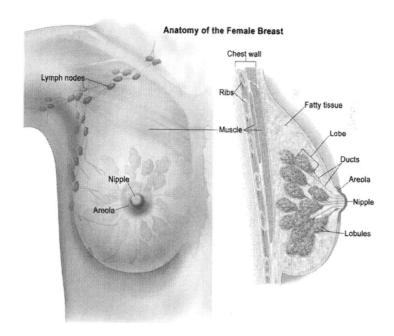

Anatomy of the Female Breast

Each woman is different, so find which one works best for you:

- Upright- Sitting up with your back straight.

- Mobile- Carrying your baby in a carrier or sling. This allows you to do other tasks while feeding.

- On your back- Sitting slightly upright. Is ideal for feeding two babies simultaneously.

- Lying down- Ideal for those who've had a C-section or for night feedings.

- On your side- Both mother and child lay on their sides.

- Hand and Knees- This position isn't recommended normally, and involves the mother getting on all fours with the baby beneath her.

Chapter 5

Your Nursing Area

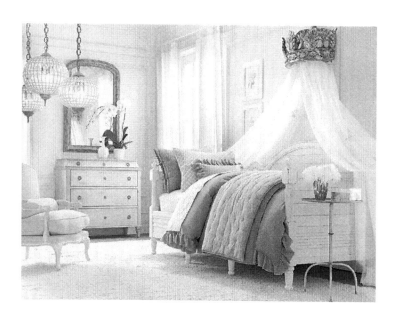

Though you might have stocked up on breast pads and nursing bras, it's also important to get your nursing area ready. It should reflect your style and be as comfortable as possible. For instance, if you prefer more quite surroundings, choose a corner in your bedroom to place a rocking chair to sit in while nursing.

However, if you would like to be in the midst of things while breastfeeding; pick a comfy armchair in the living room as your nursing spot.

Remember to take deep, calming breaths before and during breastfeeding, as it will help you to produce milk more efficiently. Also, when it comes to your nursing chair, choose one that offers good back and shoulder support. To avoid backaches, make sure you elevate your legs and feet with either a foot stool or some pillows.

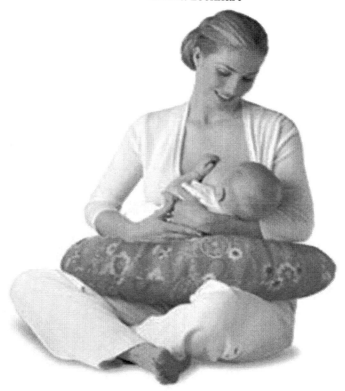

There are a few essentials that every nursing area should have. The more pillows the better, as they will provide you with much needed support and comfort during feeding times. Using pillows on your lap to support the baby is a great idea, as well. There are even pillows on the market today which are created specifically for nursing, that encircle your waist.

Also, keep a small table beside you, as you should keep drinks and healthy snacks at the ready while you're nursing. You'll need to refuel your body as you are giving your vital nutrients to your baby.

And, last but not least, while you are breastfeeding you should have plenty of distractions on hand, because nursing sessions can last for quite a while if your baby is hungry. Have a crossword puzzle or magazine beside you, just in case you should get bored.

Things to Avoid While Breastfeeding

In order to ensure that your baby receives enough nutrition for your milk, you must ensure that you are eating a diet rich in nutrients and high in calories. Otherwise, your breast milk will be lacking in many essential vitamins.

Smoking should be avoided at all costs, as more than 20 cigarettes a day can cause diarrhea, rapid heart rate, and restlessness in infants, and can even increase the chances of sudden infant death syndrome if the baby is exposed to the smoke.

Drinking alcohol should also be limited or avoided completely, as it can cause irritability and sleeplessness in the infant. If you should have a drink, then wait 2 hours between consumption and nursing. Caffeine is another element which should be curbed, and a nursing mother should not drink more than a cup or two a day, if even that.

This stage of your baby's life is crucial, so it's best to avoid the above mentioned elements, in order to ensure the safety and health of your child.

Chapter 6

Foods to Avoid While Breastfeeding

There are certain foods which are best to avoid while you're breastfeeding. Things like chocolate, citrus fruits, spices, chili, lime, garlic, and fruits that have laxative properties are the most common foods that can upset your baby's system. However, you may find that some of these foods don't affect you or your baby, whatsoever, and that your newborn actually likes the flavor that they add to your breast milk.

There is no need to pump then dump your breast milk, as long as you avoid consuming large quantities of alcohol or are advised to dump pumped milk by your doctor, due to medications that you are taking which may affect the baby.

What To Do If You Believe That You Have A Poor Milk Supply

Though many women might fear that they will not produce enough breast milk for their baby, this is usually not the case. In most instances, simply repositioning the baby and getting them to properly latch can solve your breastfeeding problems.

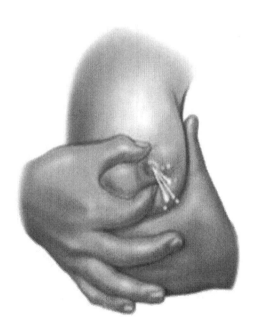

If you are preventing your child from feeding as long as they would like, due to the fact that you are concerned with not having enough breast milk, there are some simple signs to look out for to make sure that they are getting the nutrition that they need.

There are times when you're baby might seem hungry or irritable after a feeding, though these are not definite signs of hunger. The two things you should be concerned about are slow weight gain and inability to pass concentrated urine, as they are the true signs of a baby not getting enough nutritious breast milk, and you should consult with your lactation consultant or doctor.

If you are worried about your milk supply, there are a few possible ways to remedy the situation. Firstly, let your baby feed for as long as they want, as newborns will only eat if they are hungry.

Also, make sure you feed from both breasts at each sitting, and offer more feeds if your baby is not drinking enough during each feed. In addition, make sure your baby is latching properly, and that you wake them for regular feedings if they sleep for longer than 4 hours at a time.

It is normal for all babies to lose weight during their first few days of life, as they are born with stores of fat and fluids which can sustain them for that period of time. They should return back to their birth weight within a few weeks, and they will continue to put on roughly 200g for about the first four months.

Chapter 7

When You Should Use A Breast Pump

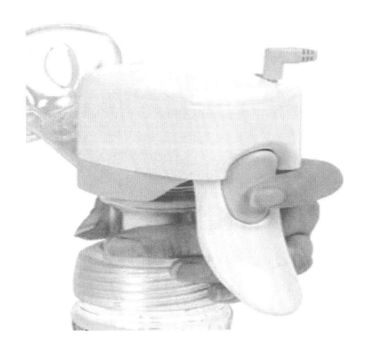

Most nursing women find that breast pumps are a convenient and highly effective way to expel and store their milk for later use, as there are many times when a mother cannot be near her child and still wants for them to get the benefits of mother's milk. There are different varieties of breast pumps.

Dual-action pumps are usually used in the hospital and are often available to rent, while smaller battery operated or hand pump units are sold in stores for general home use.

Breast pumps are ideal for working mothers, or for those who are on medications or have infections as a temporary way to express your milk and keep up your supply, without passing any harmful elements on to the baby.

Chapter 8

How To Use A Breast Pump

The benefits of extended breastfeeding have already been highlighted. However, though you may be able to physically breastfeed every time your newborn is hungry now, there may be times later down the line when it won't be so convenient.

Expressing milk to use later can free up much of your time, and prevent you from having to breastfeed in public if you'd prefer not to. By using a pump, you can provide your child with nutritious mother's milk without actually being there with them.

Learning to use a breast pump can be a bit challenging for the new mother, especially if you've already tried and were only able to express just a small amount. It will get better, don't worry. Soon you're bound to have enough milk to last for days on end.

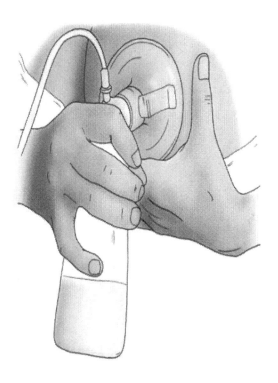

There is a certain method to the madness when it comes to breast pumps though, so here is a quick walk through of how to efficiently pump your breast milk:

- Make certain that you've read the pump instructions carefully, and that you've sterilized each part of the pump. Before the initial use, it's best to place pump elements in boiling water for at least a few minutes.

After each, thereafter, it's fine to simply wash it with hot soapy water and allow it to dry completely, unless you feel more comfortable sterilizing it after each use.

- If you've chosen an electric pump, then start off by using the lowest setting. Prepare your breasts beforehand by gently massage them and your nipples.

Keep in mind that you should relax, as this will ensure quick and proper let down.

- While you are pumping, it is often helpful to imagine yourself nursing your baby or take deep breaths in order to unwind and focus on the task at hand.

Don't get discouraged if you do not produce an adequate amount of milk, as it will most likely take a few tries to get used to the pump.

- If you are using a hand pump, start off with short, faster pumps, as this more closely mimics how your baby would feed. Longer more deliberate pumps will be sufficient once let down has occurred.

- Practicing for a few minutes each side per day in the beginning will allow for you to get the hang of it. You should eventually look forward to your pumping times, as they will usually be the most relaxing part of every day.

Chapter 9

Fitness While Breastfeeding

It's important that you maintain a healthy, active lifestyle while you are breastfeeding, as it will provide you with more energy and will help you lose the pregnancy weight which may be causing you discomfort.

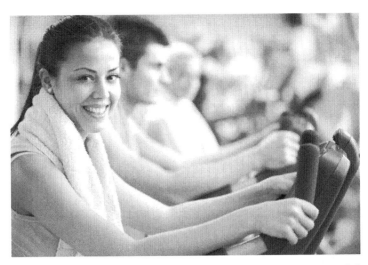

Remember to ask your doctor about how long you should wait until after giving birth to start workout, and keep in mind that a sport's bra will give you the support you need. Also, drink plenty of fluids before, during, and after your exercising.

The First Few Weeks

Breast is best, and this is especially the case with a newborn. It is the perfect food, which contains more than 400 nutrients, including hormones and compounds that will fight off disease. Your breast milk will even adjust to your baby's needs as they grow, in order to meet their dietary requirements.

It's especially important in your baby's first few weeks of life that you make sure to make yourself as comfortable as possible while nursing, as you're still new to the whole process.

Don't get too discouraged if things don't go exactly according to plan either, as it might take awhile to get the hang of it. By your first postpartum checkup you should be breastfeeding like a champ. So, enjoy the time you have with your new little one, and don't be so focused on whether or not your breastfeeding correctly, as you should really be concentrating on bonding with your baby.

Chapter 10

How to Deal With Complications that May Arise

Some breastfeeding women might experience minor problems here or there while breastfeeding. Here are a few of the most common complications that may arise and a little bit about what you should do to remedy them:

Sore Nipples

Sore nipples. A majority of nursing women will find that their nipples become sore or tender. Your nipples will usually toughen rather quickly though, so the discomfort your feeling should not last very long.

There are a number of things you can do to ease that discomfort in the meantime, however, such as:

Making sure your baby is positioned correctly, apply some high quality lanolin to your nipples after feedings, leave your breasts exposed to air for a short time after feedings (avoid covering them with fabrics right away, as this will irritate them), wash your nipples each time you breastfeed, apply teabags that have been soaked in cold water to your nipples, and change breastfeeding positions each time to avoid irritating one particular area of the nipple.

Clogged Milk Ducts

Clogged milk ducts. The signs of a clogged milk duct are small, red bumps your breast. These clogged ducts can lead to infection, so it's best to unclog them as soon as possible by making sure that you've emptied all of your milk in that breast after each feeding.

70

Offer the clogged breast to your baby first each time you breastfeed, and express the milk that is left after they're through feeding by using a breast pump. Also, make certain that your bra is not too tight, as the added pressure can exacerbate the problem.

Breast Infection (Mastitis)

Breast infection (mastitis). The symptoms of a breast infection are: pain, soreness, hardening and redness of the breast, swelling, chills, as well as heat coming from your breasts or nipples.

Mastitis is usually caused by bacteria gaining entrance to the inner breast through empty milk ducts or cracked nipples. It can also be due to a mother being overly stressed or not eating a proper diet.

Breast infections are typically treated by antibiotics, pain medications, the application of heat, plenty of rest, and getting drinking more fluids. It is also a good idea to lay in a tub of warm water as you let your breasts float, and use a hand pump to empty your milk supply.

You may think it is best to stop breastfeeding during this time, but you should not, as expressing the milk is the best thing for your healing process.

If the pain becomes too bad, then you may want to consult your doctor, as you might have an abscess. An abscess involves many of the same symptoms as mastitis, but may require more intense medications or every surgery to treat.

Refusal to Feed

Refusal to feed. If your baby is pulling away from the breast or moving his head to avoid it, then they might be suffering from an ear infection, a sore head from a vacuum delivery, or have an oral yeast infection known as thrush.

If your child is more than a few months old, they could even be teething. Yet another possible explanation is that your baby is used to dummies or nipples shield, and finds it more difficult to feed directly from the breast.

If your milk is bitter in taste, due to medications you may be taking or the fact that you are on your period, this can also be a cause of refusal to feed.

When this happens, make sure to remain patient and calm, and simply hold your baby close to you, and don't offer them the breast just yet.

Make sure that they feel safe and comfortable, and see if they nurse at the breast on their own before giving it another attempt. Also, if your baby is older, they will most likely drink less more often, so nurse only when they are ready.

Chapter 11

Starting Solid Foods

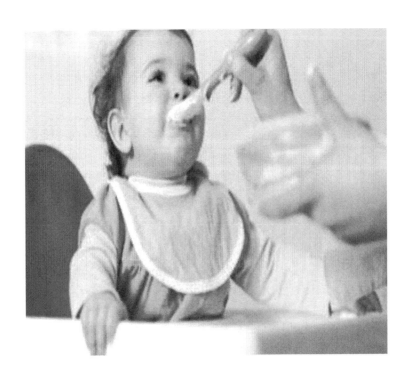

Starting solids is a big milestone for your baby. Breastfeeding is the only source of nutrition your baby will need until at least 4 months of age.

Usually full term infants will require other food sources to receive the iron they need by the time they are about 6 months old. If you are choosing to save the solids until your baby is a year old, then keep in mind that most infants at that age have more of a difficulty accepting solids.

If your child is more than 4 months old showing an interest in the food that you're eating, then it's probably a good time to start solids. However, there are cases where infants are not gaining as much weight as they should by their third month or are constantly hungry, and doctors might recommend starting solids earlier than usual.

Breastfed babies have a bit of a head start when it comes to solids, as they have already tasted a wide variety of foods via your breast milk. In addition, they will be able to digest solids better, due to the fact that breast milk contains enzymes which help to break down proteins and carbohydrates.

Your baby's first foods should be rather bland. However, they should not be spicy, and you should avoid feeding them foods which have a high risk of being allergenic. Don't be too concerned with how much your baby is eating during the introduction stage, as it is more of about experience for them, rather than receiving adequate nutrition, as you are still supplying them with breast milk.

Chapter 12

How To Wean From Breastfeeding

The weaning process can be a long and difficult one, as well as an emotional time for both you and your child. Your infant is considered weaned when they are getting all of their necessary nutrition from sources other than your breast milk and the process can take some patience if your child is not exactly ready to wean just yet.

There's no set time when you should begin to wean, as it is a matter of preference and readiness, though most believe that at roughly one year of age a child is ready to wean. You must keep in mind that it doesn't mean the end of the bond you have with your child, just that your bond will be strengthened in other ways than breastfeeding.

Weaning should be done slowly, no matter how old your infant is. To end breastfeeding too abruptly may cause trauma to your child, so it should be avoided.

Here are a few tips on how to start weaning:

- Try skipping a feeding. By offering your child a cup of juice or milk instead, or maybe even some of your pumped breast milk, you are easing your child into the transition from breastfeeding to solids. If they are older, then offer them a before bedtime snack.

- Cut your breast feedings short. If you usually nurse for twenty minutes, then make it ten from now on, as this will help your child adjust to the change slowly.

- Postponing the breast feedings. If your child typically feeds three times a day, then put the next feeding off for as long as you can, then distract the child when the specified breastfeeding time rolls around. This way, you can at least cut out a feeding or two per day.

Chapter 13

How to Lose Weight after Pregnancy

Fast Fitness Tips to Help Get You Going

Overall fitness isn't just about cardio. Although cardio is a major component of weight loss and heart health, it is important to incorporate strength training into your fitness regimen.

Strength training builds muscle mass and helps you burn more calories post-workout. Follow these strength-training tips to ramp up your workout and get a complete workout.

You shouldn't train with a weight belt. Not only has it been proven that over time the use of a weight belt decreases the strength of your abdominal and back muscles, but it has not been proven to decrease the rate of injury for those that use them. There is no reason for a belt.

A great fitness tip for people trying to develop their abs is to include squats and dead lifts into their routine. Studies have shown that these two exercises force you to use your core a great deal in order to maintain proper posture. Just remember to do each exercise correctly to avoid injury.

Exercise

Make exercise a game for you and your family. Get the whole family their own pedometer so they can count the number of steps they take per day.

Make a goal for each member of the family, and see who can take the most steps during the day. Make a chart logging everyone's progress, and the winner at the end of the month gets to delegate a week's worth of chores to whomever they choose!

We all know that exercise is good for our mind and body, but there are times when you need to give your body a rest. Most of the time if you listen to your body, it will tell you if it has been overworked and needs to recover.

Sometimes it's okay to skip a workout if you're feeling sick or run down, you haven't gotten enough sleep or are nursing an injury.

To build real strength, make sure you exercise your muscle groups in many different ways. Sticking with one form of exercise for a muscle group (like machine work only) can increase your strength in relation to that activity, but can actually weaken you when it comes to other activities that your body is not used to.

Losing Belly Fat Tips

If you are trying to focus on losing belly fat, do not work on your abs. Although you will gain muscle, you are not losing fat. It is okay to do sit ups and crunches but incorporate more aerobic exercises into your routine in order to lose unwanted belly fat.

You will not be able to get a six-pack by doing endless stomach exercise. Stomach exercises will reinforce your muscles; however, they won't burn-off your stubborn belly fat.

If your goal is to achieve a washboard abs, you'll need to lower your complete body fat by doing a lot of cardiovascular exercise and resistance training and improving your diet.

Strengthening your core leads to great total-body fitness. Your back and abdominal muscles support the rest of your body, and control your flexibility and power in almost every physical motion. By building muscle in your core, you also burn more calories in your midsection, and avoid the accumulation of belly fat.

Set A Weight Loss Goal

Choose your exercises and lifting programs carefully, if you are aiming at weight-loss as your ultimate goal. Certain weight-training regimens are designed to add muscle bulk to your frame or increase power-lifting and short-twitch muscles.

These exercises may actually increase your weight. To lose unwanted fat and pounds, choose exercises that build lean muscle and tone your body. Perform higher numbers of repetitions at lower weight in order to build this kind of muscle.

Walking

We do it every day, but there's a good chance that we could be doing it a lot more. Even minor adjustments in your daily number of steps can contribute to weight loss. Try parking at the end of the lot, taking the stairs instead of the elevator, or simply taking a leisurely stroll around the block.

It's a good idea to get at least 30 minutes of cardiovascular exercise every day. Not only will this lead to weight loss but it will strengthen your muscles, including your heart, as well as improve your overall health. Keep in mind, the longer your cardio session, the longer the recuperation time will be for your body.

Obviously, there are many options when it comes to working strength moves into your fitness routine. Keep doing your cardio, but additionally, choose any number of the tips mentioned to keep your muscles strong and prevent injury. Not only will you increase your calorie burn, but you'll have awesome muscle definition to boot.

Conclusion

Breastfeeding is truly one of the most wonderful and special things you can do for your child. It allows for you to bond with them in a way that is remarkable, and provide them with vital nutrients that will give them a head start in life.

It is, most assuredly, worth every bit of time and effort that you put into it. And, even if your child might never thank you for giving them this precious gift, you'll always know that you gave them the best by providing them with nature's perfect food.

About The Author

Emma Lockhart is a mother of a beautiful baby boy, who she adores daily. She has worked as a nurse for 12 years and has also been a midwife and breastfeeding counselor.

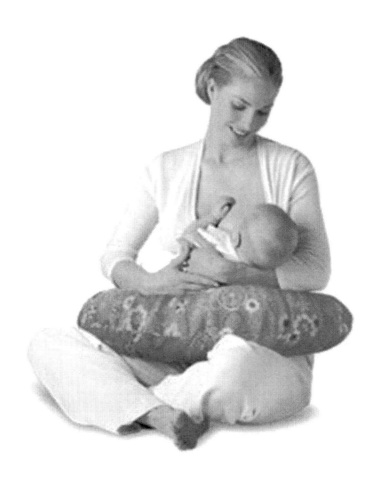

Made in the USA
Middletown, DE
07 February 2018